# PRACTICAL INSULIN
### 5TH EDITION

**A HANDBOOK FOR
PRESCRIBING PROVIDERS**

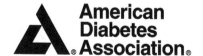

*Associate Publisher, Books,* Abe Ogden; *Director, Book Operations,* Victor Van Beuren; *Managing Editor, Books,* John Clark; *Associate Director, Book Marketing,* Annette Reape; *Acquisitions Editor,* Jaclyn Konich; *Senior Manager, Book Editing,* Lauren Wilson; *Writer,* Dr. Joshua Neumiller; *Project Manager,* Cenveo Publisher Services; *Composition,* Cenveo Publisher Services; *Cover Design,* ADA; *Printer,* Lightning Source®.

©2019 by the American Diabetes Association. All Rights Reserved. No part of this publication may be reproduced or transmitted in any form or by any means, electronic or mechanical, including duplication, recording, or any information storage and retrieval system, without the prior written permission of the American Diabetes Association.

Printed in the United States of America
1 3 5 7 9 10 8 6 4 2

The suggestions and information contained in this publication are generally consistent with the *Standards of Medical Care in Diabetes* and other policies of the American Diabetes Association, but they do not represent the policy or position of the Association or any of its boards or committees. Reasonable steps have been taken to ensure the accuracy of the information presented. However, the American Diabetes Association cannot ensure the safety or efficacy of any product or service described in this publication. Individuals are advised to consult a physician or other appropriate health care professional before undertaking any diet or exercise program or taking any medication referred to in this publication. Professionals must use and apply their own professional judgment, experience, and training and should not rely solely on the information contained in this publication before prescribing any diet, exercise, or medication. The American Diabetes Association—its officers, directors, employees, volunteers, and members—assumes no responsibility or liability for personal or other injury, loss, or damage that may result from the suggestions or information in this publication.

Jennifer Trujillo, PharmD, conducted the internal review of this book to ensure that it meets American Diabetes Association guidelines.

∞ The paper in this publication meets the requirements of the ANSI Standard Z39.48-1992 (permanence of paper).

ADA titles may be purchased for business or promotional use or for special sales. To purchase more than 50 copies of this book at a discount, or for custom editions of this book with your logo, contact the American Diabetes Association at the address below or at booksales@diabetes.org.

American Diabetes Association
2451 Crystal Drive, Suite 900
Arlington, VA 22202

DOI: 10.2337/9781580407359

**Library of Congress Cataloging-in-Publication Data**
Names: American Diabetes Association, issuing body.
Title: Practical insulin : a handbook for prescribing providers / American Diabetes Association.
Description: 5th edition. | Arlington : American Diabetes Association, [2019] | Includes bibliographical references and index.
Identifiers: LCCN 2019015901 | ISBN 9781580407359 (softcover : alk. paper)
Subjects: | MESH: Diabetes Mellitus–drug therapy | Insulin–therapeutic use | Handbook
Classification: LCC RC661.I6 | NLM WK 39 | DDC 616.4/62061–dc23
LC record available at https://lccn.loc.gov/2019015901

# Contents

**Introduction** . . . . . . . . . . . . . . . . . . . . . . . . . . . . . . . . . . . . . . . 1
**Insulin: Basic Pharmacology** . . . . . . . . . . . . . . . . . . . . . . . . . 3
**Available Insulin Products** . . . . . . . . . . . . . . . . . . . . . . . . . . 7
   Rapid-Acting Insulin. . . . . . . . . . . . . . . . . . . . . . . . . . . . . . . 7
   Short-Acting Insulin . . . . . . . . . . . . . . . . . . . . . . . . . . . . . . 11
   Intermediate-Acting Insulin . . . . . . . . . . . . . . . . . . . . . . . . 11
   Long-Acting Insulin . . . . . . . . . . . . . . . . . . . . . . . . . . . . . . 12
      Insulin Glargine (U-100) . . . . . . . . . . . . . . . . . . . . . . . . 12
      Insulin Detemir . . . . . . . . . . . . . . . . . . . . . . . . . . . . . . 12
      Insulin Glargine (U-300) . . . . . . . . . . . . . . . . . . . . . . . . 13
      Insulin Degludec (U-100; U-200) . . . . . . . . . . . . . . . . . 13
   U-500 Regular Insulin . . . . . . . . . . . . . . . . . . . . . . . . . . . 14
   Premixed Insulin Products. . . . . . . . . . . . . . . . . . . . . . . . 15
**Insulin Administration and Use Considerations** . . . . . . . . . . 17
   Insulin Delivery Method . . . . . . . . . . . . . . . . . . . . . . . . . . 17
      Vial and Syringe . . . . . . . . . . . . . . . . . . . . . . . . . . . . . 20
      Insulin Pens . . . . . . . . . . . . . . . . . . . . . . . . . . . . . . . . 20

    Continuous Subcutaneous Insulin
       Infusion (CSII; Insulin Pump)........................ 20
    Injection Technique ..................................... 22
       Factors That May Affect Absorption ................. 23
    Insulin Storage........................................ 25

**General Approaches and Recommendations for Insulin Use in People with Diabetes** ............... 27
    Type 1 Diabetes ....................................... 27
       Glycemic Treatment Goals in People
         with Type 1 Diabetes............................ 28
       Insulin Initiation and Titration ....................... 30
    Type 2 Diabetes ....................................... 33

**Sample Insulin Regimens** ............................. 37
    Two Injections per Day................................ 37
    Three Injections per Day.............................. 38
    Four Injections per Day, Regimen 1 .................. 39
    Four Injections per Day, Regimen 2 .................. 41

**Troubleshooting Barriers to Insulin Use and Key Adverse Events** ....................................... 43
    Barriers to Insulin Use in Type 2 Diabetes .............. 43
    Hypoglycemia ........................................ 44
       Hypoglycemia Unawareness ....................... 46
    Weight Gain .......................................... 46
    Adjustments for Physical Activity....................... 47

**Patient Education and Resources** ....................... 49

**Appendix 1: Typical Development and Diabetes Demands and Priorities Across Childhood** ... 51

**Appendix 2: Sample Blood Glucose Log** ................ 53

**Index** ................................................. 55

# Introduction

Joshua J. Neumiller, PharmD, CDE, FAADE, FASCP[1]

There is a good chance your practice is handling an ever-increasing number of patients with diabetes. Insulin therapy is a medical necessity for all patients with type 1 diabetes (T1D) and a useful treatment option for the many patients with type 2 diabetes (T2D) who are unable to reach individualized glycemic goals without insulin therapy. Understanding insulin products currently available on the market and current recommendations for use is vital to you and the care of your patients. Insulin's ability to lower glucose is unparalleled. Insulin both increases glucose uptake by tissues (muscle and adipose) and suppresses hepatic glucose release. The primary safety concern and limitation to insulin use is treatment-emergent hypoglycemia. In addition, insulin therapy often leads to weight gain, a negative effect for patients with T1D as well as for those with T2D who already are struggling with weight issues. In this handbook, you will find information on the many common challenges involved in managing patients on insulin—from choosing insulin regimens, to addressing patient reluctance to starting insulin therapy, to minimizing the weight gain and hypoglycemia that often accompany improved glycemic control. As is true in the general

---

[1] Vice Chair and Allen I. White Distinguished Associate Professor, Department of Pharmacotherapy, College of Pharmacy and Pharmaceutical Sciences, Washington State University, Spokane, WA.

management of diabetes, insulin therapy must be individualized to the needs and priorities of the patient, with no single insulin regimen being appropriate for all patients with diabetes. Following recommended approaches to initiating and titrating insulin therapy in consideration of individualized treatment goals and based on self-monitoring of blood glucose (SMBG) and hemoglobin $A_{1c}$ (A1C) data will help you guide the patient to achieve optimal blood glucose management while minimizing associated risks. The American Diabetes Association has published this fifth edition of *Practical Insulin: A Handbook for Prescribing Providers* in the hope that it will assist you as a clinical reference in your efforts to initiate and optimize insulin therapy for your patients with T1D and T2D.

# Insulin: Basic Pharmacology

Insulin is produced in the pancreas within the islets of Langerhans by β-cells and is secreted in response to rising blood glucose levels and neurohormonal signaling. When functioning normally, β-cells help maintain euglycemia via endogenous release of insulin to cover basal and prandial needs. In normal physiology, "basal insulin secretion" describes the low rate of insulin release between meals that is sufficient to inhibit the overproduction of glucose and ketone bodies by the liver in the fasting state. Additional bursts of insulin are released to prevent hyperglycemia in the prandial state and promote conversion of nutrients to energy for short- and long-term nutrient use and storage (see **Figure 1**). Although **Figure 1** provides generalized statements related to physiologic insulin secretion, individual responses will vary.

Insulin action involves a complex series of responses that affect carbohydrate, lipid, and protein metabolism. Insulin carries out its metabolic and growth-promoting effects by binding to insulin receptors on cell plasma membranes. A key metabolic effect of insulin receptor activation is the stimulation of glucose transport and metabolism. In the context of T1D, patients have an absolute insulin deficiency and are unable to effectively transport and metabolize glucose. In patients with T2D, the tissues are resistant to the effects of insulin, which leads to a relative deficiency in insulin release. Over time, pancreatic β-cells begin to fail in people with T2D as they continually work to produce

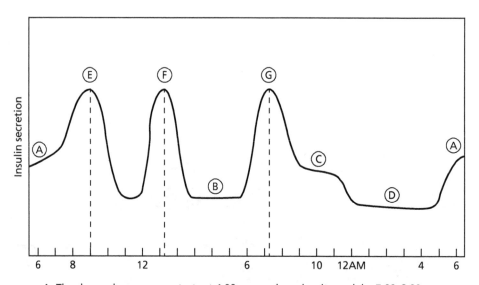

A: The dawn phenomenon starts at 4:00 A.M. and reaches its peak by 7:00–8:00 A.M. This peak is sustained until around 10:00 A.M., when levels fall. The dawn phenomenon may be a result of growth hormone and cortisol release, which begin to rise at 4:00 A.M., peak at 8:00 A.M., and fall at 10:00 A.M.

B: During the day in the fasting state, a small amount of basal insulin is released to maintain fasting glucose levels.

C: Because people are generally less active during the evening, insulin requirements tend to be slightly higher from 6:00 P.M. to 12:00 A.M. However, the increased insulin requirement is an individualized response.

D: The hormones are at their nadir from 12:00 A.M. to 4:00 A.M., so insulin requirements are lower.

E–G: Bursts of insulin are released from the pancreas to cover carbohydrate consumed with meals.

**Figure 1** — 24-h normal physiologic insulin secretion.

more insulin to counterbalance the persistent insulin resistance within the tissues. Eventually, β-cell function can decline to a level that requires exogenous insulin administration to adequately control blood glucose. Although all insulin products work through stimulation of insulin receptors, their pharmacokinetic and pharmacodynamic profiles can vary significantly. The insulin primarily in use today is manufactured by way of recombinant DNA technology as either human insulin (**Figure 2**) or as rapid- or long-acting human analogs. Analog insulins are structurally modified such that the amino acid sequence is intentionally altered to achieve desired pharmacokinetic characteristics.

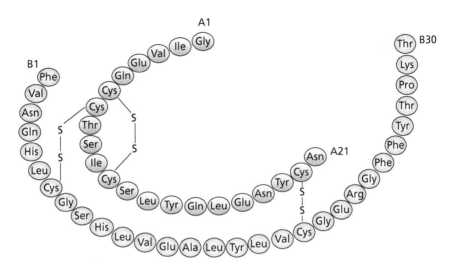

**Figure 2**—Structure of human insulin.

*Source:* Adapted from FeF Chemicals (available from www.fefchemicals.com/biopharm/scientific-information/articles/the-insulin-peptide-family).

# Available Insulin Products

Insulin potency is measured in units. Preparations sold in the U.S. at the time of this publication are available in several concentrations, including U-100 (100 units/mL), U-200 (200 units/mL), U-300 (300 units/mL), and U-500 (500 units/mL) products. U-500 insulin is generally reserved for patients with extreme insulin resistance who take large daily doses of insulin, as discussed in the section **U-500 Regular Insulin** (p. 14). **Table 1** summarizes key pharmacokinetic and pharmacodynamic properties of insulin products currently available in the U.S. The following sections discuss individual insulin products, as grouped by their action profiles. A visual representation of the time-action profiles of currently available insulin products is provided in **Figure 3**.

## Rapid-Acting Insulin

Rapid-acting insulin analogs are intended to mimic meal-stimulated insulin secretion. Their rapid onset improves our ability to match the insulin dose to carbohydrate intake and ensure that insulin and glucose reach the blood at approximately the same moment. Currently available injectable rapid-acting analogs (RAAs) include insulin lispro, insulin aspart, and insulin glulisine. RAAs are the insulin of choice for use in insulin pumps (see the section **INSULIN ADMINISTRATION AND USE CONSIDERATIONS** (p. 17) for additional information on insulin pump use). Injectable RAAs are engi-

## Table 1 — Summary of Insulin Pharmacokinetic and Pharmacodynamic Properties*

| | Product | Time to Onset of Action (h) | Time to Peak Action (h) | Duration of Action (h) |
|---|---|---|---|---|
| **Generic Name** | **Brand Name(s)** | | | |
| Regular Human Insulin (U-100) | Humulin R; Novolin R | 0.5 | 1.5–2.5 | 8 |
| Lispro (U-100, U-200) | Humalog; Admelog | within 0.25 | 0.5–1.5 | 4–6 |
| Aspart[†] | NovoLog, Fiasp | within 0.25 | 0.5–1.5 | 4–6 |
| Glulisine | Apidra | within 0.25 | 0.5–1.5 | 4–6 |
| Inhaled Human Insulin Powder | Afrezza | within 0.25 | 0.5–1 | 1.5–4.5 |
| NPH Insulin | Humulin N; Novolin N | 2–4 | 4–10 | 12–18 |
| Detemir | Levemir | 2–4 | flat | 14–24 |
| Glargine (U-100) | Lantus; Basaglar | 2–4 | flat | 20–24 |
| Glargine (U-300) | Toujeo | 6 | flat | up to 36 |
| Degludec (U-100, U-200) | Tresiba | 1 | flat | >42 |
| Regular Human Insulin (U-500) | Humulin R U-500 | 0.5 | 4–8 | 13–24 |

**Abbreviations:** h: hours.
* Person-specific onset, peak, and duration may vary from times listed in table. Peak and duration are dose dependent with shorter durations of action seen for smaller doses and longer durations of action with larger doses.
† Insulin aspart is available as two branded products: NovoLog and Fiasp. Fiasp has a relatively fast onset of action and has been shown to provide greater reductions in 1-h postprandial glucose levels compared with NovoLog.

neered to dissociate and be absorbed more rapidly than regular human insulin (RHI), resulting in a faster onset and shorter duration of action. The faster onset of action allows for RAAs to be administered closer to the time of meal ingestion (typically 15 min before a meal), and the shorter duration of action lends to a reduction in hypoglycemic events between meals. As an example, in one study, following subcutaneous (SC) administration of insulin lispro at doses ranging from 0.1–0.4 unit/kg, peak serum levels were seen within 30–90 min, compared with 50–120 min with RHI. Similar observations have been noted in studies with insulin aspart and insulin glulisine. Insulin lispro is commercially available in both U-100 and U-200 strengths, with a follow-on U-100 insulin lispro product recently approved by the U.S. Food and Drug

AVAILABLE INSULIN PRODUCTS 9

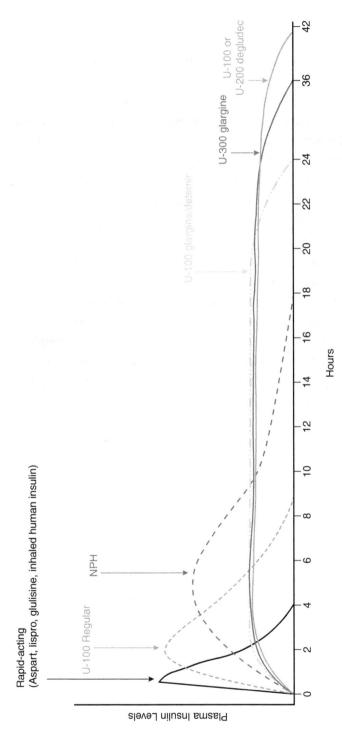

**Figure 3**—Insulin products by comparative action.

Administration (FDA) under the brand name Admelog. Notably, in 2019 the manufacturer of Humalog began producing an identical generic insulin lispro product to be sold at a reduced cost. Insulin aspart is likewise available as two different branded products: NovoLog and Fiasp. The faster acting insulin aspart product (Fiasp) is formulated with niacinamide, which is believed to promote the formation of insulin monomers after SC injection, leading to more rapid absorption. Clinical trials comparing Fiasp and NovoLog in people with T1D and T2D showed a statistically significant improvement in lowering of 1-h postprandial glucose levels with Fiasp. It is generally recommended that RAAs be administered no more than 15 min before a meal; however, it is acceptable for people to inject after a meal if carbohydrate intake is difficult to predict or if their rate of carbohydrate absorption is variable because of gastroparesis. It is possible that the faster-acting insulin aspart product (Fiasp) may have an advantage in this scenario because of its relatively rapid absorption.

The mechanism of action of inhalable human insulin powder (brand name Afrezza), also classified as an RAA, differs from the injectable rapid-acting insulins. The product is composed of insulin formulated in "microspheres" with a carrier molecule that allows for the insulin to be delivered into the deep lung for rapid absorption following inhalation (see **Figure 4**). Inhaled human insulin is approved for use in people with T1D and T2D and is a viable option for people who are unwilling to initiate SC self-injection and can benefit from prandial insulin administration. This inhaled insulin product is contraindicated

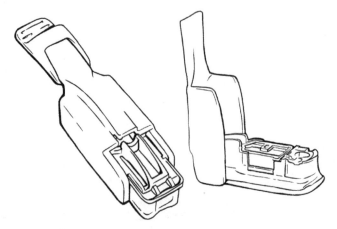

**Figure 4**—Afrezza inhaler.

in people with a chronic lung disease, such as asthma and chronic obstructive pulmonary disease, because of the risk of acute bronchospasm.

## Short-Acting Insulin

RHI generally is classified as a short-acting insulin product. Like the RAAs just discussed, RHI is a prandial (mealtime) insulin product used to cover carbohydrate intake with meals. When compared with rapid-acting insulin analogs, RHI has a slower onset and a longer duration of action (see **Table 1**). Following a single SC injection of 0.1 unit/kg of RHI to healthy subjects, peak insulin concentrations generally occur between 1.5 and 2.5 h post dose, with insulin concentrations returning to baseline after ~5 h. The glucose-lowering effect of RHI starts ~30 min after SC administration; thus, RHI is typically injected 30–45 min before a meal to best match the expected postprandial rise in blood glucose. RHI administration through continuous intravenous infusion is typically the treatment of choice for managing hyperglycemia in the critical-care setting. Although rapid-acting insulin analogs have possible advantages related to their faster onset and shorter durations of action, RHI costs considerably less and can be used effectively in patients unable to afford newer analog insulin products. Of note, RHI can be purchased without a prescription at the pharmacy. A specific Walmart brand of RHI (ReliOn) can be purchased without a prescription for approximately $30 per vial.

## Intermediate-Acting Insulin

Neutral protamine Hagedorn (NPH) insulin, also known as isophane insulin, is generally classified as "intermediate acting" in terms of its pharmacokinetic profile. NPH insulin contains an absorption-inhibiting substance called protamine, which prolongs the action and contributes to the cloudy appearance of NPH insulin. For this reason, NPH and NPH-type insulins (such as those contained in premixed insulin products) should be agitated or mixed before injection to resuspend the insulin mixture. NPH insulin may be used to cover basal insulin needs, in which case NPH is typically administered twice daily. NPH reaches peak plasma levels anywhere from 4–10 h after SC administration (see **Table 1**). Because of the notable peak with NPH insulin, its use is associated with higher rates of hypoglycemia compared with long-acting insulin analogs. Although NPH does carry a higher hypoglycemia risk, it is considerably less expensive than long-acting insulin analogs and can be used effectively in people who have difficulty obtaining more expensive insulin products. As discussed above for RHI, NPH insulin can be purchased without a prescription. Walmart also sells NPH insulin (ReliOn) without a prescription for approximately $30 per vial.

## Long-Acting Insulin

Long-acting insulin products are basal insulin analogs that provide basal insulin coverage for up to 24 h or longer, depending on the product.

### Insulin Glargine (U-100)

Insulin glargine (U-100) differs structurally from human insulin by the addition of two arginines after position B30 and the replacement of asparagine with glycine at position A21. Unlike NPH insulin, insulin glargine is soluble at a pH of 4.0. Following SC injection, the acidic insulin solution is neutralized, leading to the formation of insulin microprecipitates from which small amounts of insulin are gradually released over time. As noted in **Table 1**, U-100 insulin glargine exhibits a duration of action generally ranging from 20–24 h with a relatively flat pharmacokinetic profile. In clinical trials, U-100 insulin glargine demonstrated similar effects on glycemic control when compared to once- or twice-daily NPH, with the advantage of a decreased rate of hypoglycemic events, particularly nocturnal hypoglycemic events. In addition to the insulin glargine product Lantus, a follow-on U-100 insulin glargine product is available in the U.S., marketed as Basaglar. Although some people can realize a full 24 h of basal coverage with a single injection of U-100 insulin glargine, some people require twice-daily administration for a full 24 h of basal coverage.

### Insulin Detemir

Insulin detemir is another long-acting basal insulin analog. Insulin detemir has a prolonged duration of action (14–24 h) because of its ability to reversibly bind to albumin at the injection site and within the bloodstream. Structurally, insulin detemir differs from human insulin by the omission of threonine at position B30 and the attachment of myristic acid to lysine at position B29. The presence of myristic acid contributes to delayed dissociation and absorption of insulin detemir hexamers and facilitates a >98% binding of insulin detemir to albumin in the plasma and interstitial fluid. Because only free, non-albumin-bound insulin can be absorbed, albumin binding contributes to the prolonged duration of action seen with insulin detemir. Because the duration of action of insulin detemir can range from 14–24 h, not everyone can realize a full 24 h of basal insulin coverage with once-daily administration. Twice-daily administration may be required in some patients.

### Insulin Glargine (U-300)

U-300 insulin glargine is a threefold concentrated version of insulin glargine. U-300 insulin glargine is similar to the U-100 product in terms of structure and solubility at an acidic pH of 4.0. The longer duration of action realized with the concentrated U-300 product is attributable to the smaller injection volume, which results in a smaller precipitate surface area. The smaller surface area results in a slower dissolution rate and a resultant longer duration of action (see **Figure 3**). Although the U-100 version of insulin glargine requires twice-daily administration in some patients to achieve a full 24 h of basal coverage, once-daily administration of U-300 insulin glargine is sufficient to provide a full day of basal coverage given its longer duration of action. Because of the pharmacokinetic and pharmacodynamic properties of U-300 insulin glargine, time is needed for this insulin product to accumulate and reach steady-state levels, which generally are achieved after 5 days of once-daily administration. The manufacturer recommends titrating the dose no more frequently than every 3–4 days to minimize the risk of hypoglycemia.

Potential advantages of U-300 insulin glargine over the U-100 insulin glargine product include a longer duration of action, the potential for delivery of large insulin doses in a smaller injection volume, and a lower incidence of nocturnal hypoglycemia. Of note, when converting someone from the U-100 insulin glargine product to the U-300 product, larger doses (on a unit-per-unit basis) are typically needed to achieve the same glucose-lowering effect. Therefore, it can be expected that higher unit doses of U-300 insulin glargine will be required to maintain glycemic control compared with the previous U-100 insulin glargine dose.

### Insulin Degludec (U-100; U-200)

Insulin degludec is another long-acting basal insulin analog with a duration of action in excess of 42 h. Like U-300 insulin glargine, a single daily dose of insulin degludec will always provide sufficient coverage for a full 24 h. Steady-state insulin concentrations are achieved by 3–4 days of once-daily SC administration. To achieve this prolonged glycemic effect, insulin degludec is modified such that the amino acid at B30 is deleted and the lysine at position B29 is conjugated to hexadecanoic acid. When stored in solution with phenol and zinc, insulin degludec forms small, soluble, and stable dihexamers. Upon injection, the phenol component slowly dissipates, allowing for self-association of the insulin molecules into large multihexameric chains consisting of thousands of dihexamers connected to one another. Over time, these chains slowly begin to dissolve as the zinc component diffuses, resulting in the release of insulin from the terminal ends of the chain to be absorbed. Insulin degludec is commercially available in U-100 and U-200 concentrations. Unlike insulin glargine, variation in the concentration of insulin degludec does not alter its pharmacokinetic and pharmacodynamic properties. Thus, differences in the duration of action are not seen when comparing the U-100 and U-200 products. Similar to U-300 insulin glargine, the manufacturer recommends titrating the dose no more frequently than every 3–4 days to minimize the risk of hypoglycemia. Potential advantages of insulin degludec include its long duration of action, the potential for delivery of large insulin doses in a smaller injection volume (U-200 product), and a lower incidence of nocturnal hypoglycemia compared with U-100 insulin glargine. In addition, insulin degludec can be particularly useful in patients with erratic schedules who may benefit from flexible dosing. Studies with insulin degludec have shown that dosing at variable times during the day has no impact on efficacy or hypoglycemia risk. It is recommended, however, that doses be separated by at least 8 h.

## U-500 Regular Insulin

U-500 regular insulin was first introduced in the U.S. in 1952 for use in people with extreme insulin resistance caused by antibody formation against animal-derived insulin products. Although a five-times concentrated RHI product, the pharmacokinetics of U-500 insulin are considerably different from U-100 RHI. U-500 insulin peaks around 30 min after SC injection and has a duration of action that can range widely (see **Table 1**). Historically, U-500 insulin use was associated with a high risk of insulin overdose errors because of injection of U-500 with U-100 insulin syringes. In recent years, however, the availability of U-500 insulin pens and dedicated U-500 insulin syringes has improved the safety of this insulin product. Given the unique properties of U-500 insulin, its use is generally reserved for people with T2D with significant insulin resistance who take in excess of 200 units of insulin daily. Following the publication of a U-500 clinical trial that used two dosing algorithms for the initiation and titration of U-500 in people with T2D who had not achieved adequate glycemic control with high-dose U-100 insulin therapy, dosing algorithms are now readily available to help guide clinicians in the use of U-500 insulin in appropriate patients.

## Premixed Insulin Products

Some insulin products can be combined, or "mixed," in the same syringe to reduce the number of required daily injections. NPH or NPH-type insulin can be mixed with either RHI or rapid-acting insulin analogs. By mixing NPH-type insulins with regular insulin or a rapid-acting insulin analog, a biphasic action profile is created, providing both basal and prandial coverage with a single injection. When mixing insulins in a single syringe, the rapid- or short-acting insulin should be drawn up first. Note that long-acting insulins, such as insulin glargine, insulin detemir, and insulin degludec, should never be mixed with other insulin products by patients in the same syringe.

Commercially available premixed insulin products contain set percentages of two types of insulins in the same solution. These include mixtures of NPH and RHI (70/30), mixtures of protamine suspensions of RAAs with the respective RAA (75/25 lispro protamine/insulin lispro, 50/50 lispro protamine/insulin lispro, and 70/30 aspart protamine/insulin aspart), and a combination of insulin degludec with insulin aspart (70/30). The primary advantages of these insulin products include convenience and accuracy of administration, particularly for people with vision or dexterity limitations for whom mixing insulin would be difficult or unreliable. In addition to fixed-dose insulin combination products, two currently available products combine a basal insulin analog with a glucagon-like peptide 1 (GLP-1) receptor agonist. Combination therapy with basal insulin and a GLP-1 receptor agonist can effectively target both fasting and postprandial glucose values and thus improve A1C and overall glycemic control while also mitigating insulin-associated weight gain. **Table 2** provides a summary of fixed-dose combination products available in the U.S. at the time of publication of this handbook.

## Table 2 – Fixed-Dose Combination Insulin Products

| Product | | | | | |
|---|---|---|---|---|---|
| Generic Name | Brand Name(s) | Product Availability | Units per Pen | Dose Range per Injection (pens only) | Recommended Pen Storage at Room Temperature (days) |
| *Fixed-Dose Combination Insulin Products* | | | | | |
| Regular/NPH 70/30 | Humulin 70/30<br>Novolin 70/30 | Vial, Prefilled pen | 300 units | 1–60 | 10 |
| Lispro mix 50/50 | Humalog Mix 50/50 | Vial, Prefilled pen | 300 units | 1–60 units | 10 |
| Lispro mix 75/25 | Humalog Mix 75/25 | Vial, Prefilled pen | 300 units | 1–60 units | 10 |
| Aspart mix 70/30 | NovoLog Mix 70/30 | Vial, Prefilled pen | 300 units | 1–60 units | 14 |
| Degludec/aspart mix 70/30 | Ryzodeg 70/30 | Prefilled pen | 300 units | 1–80 units | 28 |
| *Fixed-Dose Insulin/GLP-1 Receptor Agonist Products* | | | | | |
| Insulin Glargine/ Lixisenatide | Soliqua | Prefilled pen | 300 units (insulin glargine) | 15–60 units (insulin glargine) | 28 |
| Insulin Degludec/ Liraglutide | Xultophy | Prefilled pen | 300 units (insulin degludec) | 10–50 units (insulin degludec) | 21 |

**Abbreviations:** GLP-1: glucagon-like peptide-1.

# Insulin Administration and Use Considerations

When selecting an insulin regimen for a person with diabetes, there are a variety of factors to consider. Such factors include, but are not limited to: cost, self-management capabilities, and patient-specific treatment goals. On a product level, individual insulin products are available in different delivery devices and have different recommendations for storage and use. **Table 3** provides a summary of current insulin product availability and storage recommendations from the manufacturers. This section will discuss several insulin use considerations, including the selection of an insulin delivery method, injection technique, and insulin storage.

## Insulin Delivery Method

A variety of insulin delivery options are available. Options, in order of increasing cost of use, include use of insulin vials and syringes (**Figure 5**), pens with disposable cartridges, prefilled disposable pens (**Figure 6**), and insulin pumps. The patient's resources as well as ability to prepare and inject each insulin dose should be considered when recommending a delivery method. The American Diabetes Association (the Association) makes the following recommendations regarding use of insulin syringes and insulin pens:

- For people with diabetes who require insulin, insulin syringes or insulin pens may be used for insulin delivery with consideration of

## Table 3 — Insulin Product Availability and Storage Information

| Product | | | Units per Pen (if applicable) | Dose Range per Injection (pens only) | Recommended Pen Storage at Room Temperature (days) |
|---|---|---|---|---|---|
| Generic Name | Brand Name(s) | Product Availability | | | |
| *Prandial (Mealtime) Insulin Products* | | | | | |
| Regular Human Insulin | Humulin R, Novolin R | Vial | N/A | N/A | N/A |
| | Humulin R U-500 | Vial, Prefilled pen | 1,500 units | 5–300 units | 28 |
| Insulin Lispro | Humalog (U-100) | Vial, Prefilled pen, Pen cartridges | 300 units | 1–60 units | 28 |
| | Admelog (U-100) | Vial, Prefilled pen | 300 units | 1–80 units | 28 |
| | Humalog (U-200) | Prefilled pen | 600 units | 1–60 units | 28 |
| Insulin Aspart | NovoLog | Vial, Prefilled pen, Pen cartridges | 300 units | 1–60 units (FlexPen) 1–80 units (FlexTouch) | 28 |
| | Fiasp | Vial, Prefilled pen | 300 units | 1–80 units | 28 |
| Insulin Glulisine | Apidra | Vial, Prefilled pen | 300 units | 1–80 units | 28 |
| Inhaled Human Insulin | Afrezza | Inhalation cartridges | N/A | N/A | N/A |
| *Basal Insulin Products* | | | | | |
| Human Insulin Isophane (NPH) | Humulin N, Novolin N | Vial, Prefilled pen | 300 units | 1–60 units | 14 |
| Insulin Detemir | Levemir | Vial, Prefilled pen | 300 units | 1–80 units | 42 |
| Insulin Glargine (U-100) | Lantus | Vial, Prefilled pen | 300 units | 1–80 units | 28 |
| | Basaglar | Prefilled pen | 300 units | 1–80 units | 28 |
| Insulin Glargine (U-300) | Toujeo | Prefilled pen | 450 units (SoloStar) 900 units (Max SoloStar) | 1–80 units (SoloStar) 2–160 units (Max SoloStar) | 42 |
| Insulin Degludec (U-100, U-200) | Tresiba | Vial (U-100 only), Prefilled pen | 300 units (U-100) 600 units (U-200) | 1–80 units (U-100) 2–160 (U-200) | 56 |

**Abbreviations:** N/A: not applicable.

INSULIN ADMINISTRATION AND USE CONSIDERATIONS 19

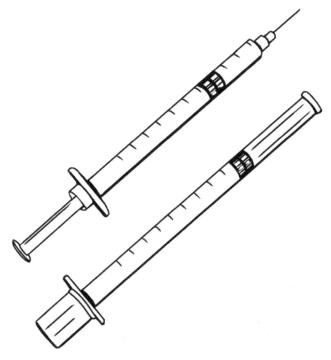

**Figure 5**—Insulin syringe.

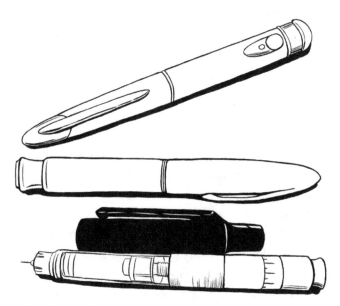

**Figure 6**—Prefilled disposable insulin pens.

patient preference, insulin type and dosing regimen, cost, and self-management capabilities.
- Insulin pens or insulin injection aids may be considered for patients with dexterity issues or vision impairment to facilitate the administration of accurate insulin doses.

## Vial and Syringe

Vials of insulin are typically less expensive than prefilled insulin pens or insulin cartridges. Many people can do quite well with vials and syringes, but use may be difficult for people with vision or dexterity issues. People should be instructed to use a new, clean needle for every dose to prevent injection site infections. Insulin syringes are available in the U.S. for U-100 and U-500 insulin products. To prevent dosing and administration errors, U-200 and U-300 insulin products are available in pens only (see **Table 3**).

## Insulin Pens

Insulin pens provide a mode of delivery that is more convenient, and often more accurate, than insulin administration using a vial and syringe. These pens can be beneficial for people who have vision or dexterity issues that make the accuracy of drawing insulin into a syringe difficult. To prevent infection, a new disposable pen needle should be tightened on to the insulin pen before each use. Some of the pens also require priming the pen needle before each use and holding the needle in the injection site for a specific number of seconds, so manufacturer instructions should be explained to the patient before initiation.

## Continuous Subcutaneous Insulin Infusion (CSII; Insulin Pump)

Motivated patients with T1D who are performing multiple daily injections (MDIs) and who desire flexibility to compensate for unscheduled activities may be candidates for continuous subcutaneous insulin infusion (CSII) through the use of an insulin pump. Most currently available insulin pumps deliver rapid-acting insulin through an SC cannula fed through tubing from the insulin pump (see **Figure 7**), while a few devices attach directly to the skin. Newer insulin pumps have the additional capability of interfacing with a continuous glucose monitor (CGM) to automate insulin delivery. Currently, CSII is largely limited to people with T1D because of limitations of insulin volume that can be loaded into an insulin pump. That said, insulin pumps are increasingly being used in the setting of T2D with the arrival of the V-Go patch pump that can deliver 24 h of

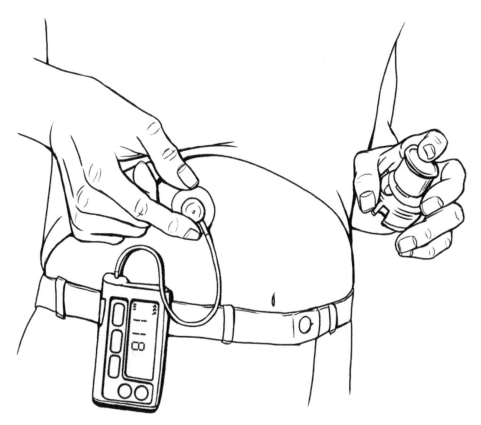

**Figure 7**—Insulin pump.

insulin to people with T2D. CSII requires considerable patient education and support until the individual becomes familiar with use of the device. Patients initiating pump therapy should be referred for diabetes education sessions with a healthcare team that is experienced in pump therapy. The Association offers the following general recommendations related to the use of insulin pumps:

- Most adults, children, and adolescents with T1D should be treated with intensive insulin therapy with either MDIs or an insulin pump.
- Insulin pump therapy may be considered as an option for all children and adolescents, especially in children under 7 years of age.
- Automated insulin delivery systems may be considered in children (>7 years) and adults with T1D to improve glycemic control.

Insulin pumps utilize rapid-acting insulin (insulin lispro, insulin aspart, or insulin glulisine) to cover both basal and bolus insulin needs (**Figure 8**).

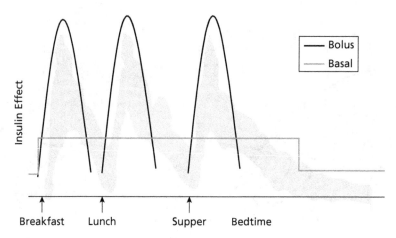

**Figure 8**—Insulin administration via an insulin pump.

Insulin pump and patch technology advances quickly, with new-generation devices entering the market regularly. The Association's publication *Diabetes Forecast* publishes consumer guides, including an insulin pump consumer guide, on an annual basis that are readily accessible on the publication website (www.diabetesforecast.org).

## Injection Technique

Ensuring that patients and caregivers understand correct insulin injection technique is important to optimize glucose control and insulin use safety. Thus, it is important that insulin be delivered into the proper tissue in the right way. Recommendations have been published elsewhere outlining best practices for insulin injection. Proper insulin injection technique includes injecting into appropriate body areas, injection site rotation, appropriate care of injection sites to avoid infection or other complications, and avoidance of intramuscular (IM) insulin delivery.

Exogenous-delivered insulin should be injected into SC tissue, not into an IM site. Recommended sites for insulin injection include the abdomen, thigh, buttock, and upper arm (**Figure 9**). Because insulin absorption from IM sites differs according to the activity of the muscle, inadvertent IM injection can lead to unpredictable insulin absorption and variable effects on glucose, with IM injection being associated with frequent and unexplained hypoglycemia in several reports. Risk for IM insulin delivery is increased in younger and lean

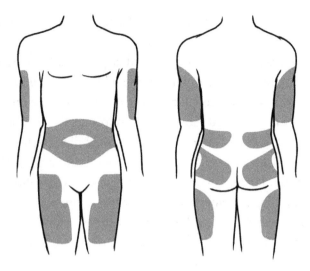

**Figure 9** — Insulin injection sites.

patients, when injecting into the limbs rather than truncal sites (abdomen and buttocks), and when using longer needles. Recent evidence supports the use of short needles (e.g., 4-mm pen needles) as being effective and well tolerated compared with longer needles, including a study performed in obese adults. Injection site rotation is also necessary to avoid lipohypertrophy and lipoatrophy. Lipohypertrophy can contribute to erratic insulin absorption and increased glycemic variability and unexplained hypoglycemic episodes. Patients or caregivers should receive education about proper injection site rotation and learn to recognize and avoid areas of lipohypertrophy. Examination of insulin injection sites for the presence of lipohypertrophy, as well as assessment of injection device use and injection technique, are key components of a comprehensive diabetes medical evaluation and treatment plan. Numerous evidence-based insulin delivery recommendations have been published. Adherence to recommendations may lead to more effective use of this therapy and, as such, may hold the potential for improved clinical outcomes.

### *Factors That May Affect Absorption*

Several factors affect the pharmacokinetic properties of insulin, regardless of insulin type. The site of injection, thickness of the SC tissue, amount of total body adipose tissue, SC blood flow, and amount of insulin administered all can affect the pharmacokinetics of exogenous insulin. Factors such as level of endogenous insulin secretion (T1D versus T2D) and obesity also may contribute to pharmacokinetic differences observed among individual patients. Temperature variation can have a major influence on insulin absorption. Elevated skin temperature can lead to increased SC vasodilation, increasing blood flow to the injection site and causing insulin to be absorbed more rapidly. Additionally, SC injections can be administered at multiple anatomic sites, such as the abdominal wall area, thigh, or upper arm. Most insulin manufacturers recommend rotating injection sites, but changing the anatomic site of injection can affect insulin absorption. People using insulin should be educated about factors that may influence insulin absorption when initiating insulin therapy and periodically thereafter.

The following factors may be considered to facilitate more predictable absorption:

- **Injection site:** Potential SC injection sites include the abdomen (avoiding 1–2 inches around the navel), upper thighs, hips and buttocks, or back of the upper arms. However, injections into the abdomen, with its larger overall blood circulation and higher body heat, provide the quickest and most predictable absorption of rapid-acting and regular insulin. Avoidance of edematous sites is advisable.
- **Injection site rotation:** Patients can choose one body area for injection and rotate within that area or can rotate among body areas. Systematic rotation prevents lipohypertrophy, a result of insulin stimulation of fat cell growth, which delays insulin absorption. If patients develop sites of lipohypertrophy, they should avoid injecting into these areas.
- **Injection volume:** Variability in insulin absorption is increased and net absorption is decreased as the volume of insulin in a single injection increases. For patients with significant insulin resistance who are using large doses of insulin, smaller injections given multiple times per day may help decrease the variability in absorption. Using concentrated insulin products is another approach that may decrease injection volume.
- **Blood flow:** Practices that increase regional blood flow (e.g., exercise, local massage or friction, hot showers, or soaks and saunas) can speed the absorption of insulin and thus alter insulin action.

## Insulin Storage

Unopened vials, cartridges, and pens of insulin should be refrigerated when not in use and should be used before the expiration date. Once opened, insulin vials should be stored at room temperature. While in use, insulin pens should never be stored with a pen needle attached to prevent contamination of the insulin. Encourage patients to follow the manufacturer's recommendations for storing open insulin pens or cartridges (see **Table 2** and **Table 3**).

Exposure to freezing, direct sunlight, or high temperatures will decrease insulin potency. Instruct patients to examine insulin appearance before injection. NPH insulin should appear uniformly cloudy without clumping or sediment after gentle resuspension; rapid-, short-, and long-acting insulins should appear clear without any particulates in the insulin solution. Counsel patients not to use insulin if the appearance is not correct and to contact their pharmacist or provider for further advice.

# General Approaches and Recommendations for Insulin Use in People with Diabetes

Among all available glucose-lowering strategies, intensive (basal/bolus) insulin therapy has the greatest potential for lowering A1C and improving glycemic control. The degree to which glycemia can be reduced with intensive insulin therapy is limited only by hypoglycemia. Unlike many other antihyperglycemic options that target either fasting plasma glucose or postprandial glucose, insulin can be used to target fasting glucose, postprandial glucose, or both, depending on the needs of the individual. Given the risks of hypoglycemia and weight gain, however, the risks and benefits of insulin treatment must be considered against those of other treatment approaches in people with T2D.

The following sections provide a general description of the approaches to insulin use in people with T1D and T2D. Although this information may be helpful in understanding the generally recommended approaches to insulin use in these patient populations, the information provided is by no means the only approach to successfully managing diabetes with insulin.

## Type 1 Diabetes

Exogenous insulin therapy is a requirement for people with T1D because of an absolute lack of endogenous insulin secretion from pancreatic β-cells. As such, all people with T1D should be managed with an intensive insulin regimen designed to cover both basal and prandial (mealtime) insulin needs, with the ultimate goal of achieving individualized glycemic goals. Indeed, the Diabetes Control and Complications Trial (DCCT) showed that intensive therapy with MDIs or CSII resulted in improved glycemic control and better long-term outcomes in people with T1D. The Association makes the following specific recommendations pertaining to insulin therapy in people with T1D:

- Most people with T1D should be treated with MDIs of prandial insulin and basal insulin or CSII.
- Most individuals with T1D should use rapid-acting insulin analogs to reduce hypoglycemia risk.
- Individuals with T1D should be educated on matching prandial insulin doses to carbohydrate intake, premeal blood glucose levels, and anticipated physical activity.

Ideally the exogenous insulin regimen used in people with T1D mimics physiologic insulin secretory patterns to the extent possible. Such an approach involves either initiation of an intensive MDI insulin regimen or use of CSII. An intensive basal/bolus regimen in someone with T1D is generally inclusive of a long-acting insulin that mimics normal basal insulin release seen in people without diabetes in which ~1 unit of insulin is secreted every hour to handle the fasting insulin needs of the liver and muscle. A rapid-acting insulin is also administered in conjunction with the ingestion of carbohydrates at mealtimes, which simulates the rapid release of insulin from the pancreas that typically occurs in the fed state. Similarly, CSII allows for the infusion of rapid-acting insulin to cover both basal and prandial insulin needs (**Figure 8**).

## Glycemic Treatment Goals in People with Type 1 Diabetes

As noted previously, treatment goals and expectations should be individualized for all people with diabetes, including those with T1D. Aside from the importance of individualization, major organizations, including the American Diabetes Association, recommend different general treatment targets for children and adolescents compared with adults with T1D. **Table 4** summarizes general glycemic recommendations for nonpregnant adults with diabetes, and **Table 5** summarizes general glycemic goals for children and adolescents with T1D. Note that although general recommendations for A1C and blood glucose levels are provided, all glycemic goals should be individualized based on person-specific considerations. Factors that may inform glycemic goals in an

## Table 4—Glycemic Recommendations for Many Nonpregnant Adults with Diabetes

| A1C | <7.0%* |
|---|---|
| Fasting (Preprandial) Glucose | 80–130 mg/dL* |
| Postprandial Glucose | <180 mg/dL* |

*More or less stringent goals may be appropriate for individuals.

## Table 5—Glycemic Goals for Children and Adolescents with Type 1 Diabetes

| A1C | <7.5%* |
|---|---|
| Premeal Glucose | 90–130 mg/dL* |
| Bedtime/Overnight Glucose | 90–150 mg/dL* |

*More or less stringent goals may be appropriate for individuals.

individual may include risk of hypoglycemia and other adverse drug events, diabetes disease duration, life expectancy, comorbidity burden, presence of vascular complications, attitudes and treatment expectations of the individual, and resources and support available to implement a given treatment plan. When glycemic goal setting in children and adolescents with T1D, the Association outlines the following key considerations:

- Goals should be individualized, and lower goals may be reasonable based on a benefit-risk assessment.
- Blood glucose goals should be modified in children with frequent hypoglycemia or hypoglycemia unawareness.
- Postprandial blood glucose values should be measured when there is a discrepancy between preprandial blood glucose values and A1C levels and to assess preprandial insulin doses in those on basal/bolus or CSII regimens.

Ultimately, the Association recommends that treatment decisions and glycemic goal setting should be made in collaboration with the individual, whenever possible, to incorporate his or her needs, preferences, and values.

## Insulin Initiation and Titration

When initiating insulin therapy in someone newly diagnosed with T1D, the starting insulin dose is generally calculated based on weight, with starting doses typically ranging from 0.4–1.0 unit/kg/day of total insulin. Many clinicians will begin at 0.5 unit/kg/day when the person is metabolically stable, with subsequent titration of the insulin per glycemic response. After calculating the total daily insulin dose, approximately half of the calculated total daily dose is administered as basal insulin, with the other half distributed across meals as prandial insulin (such as one-sixth of the total daily dose injected at breakfast, lunch, and dinner, as an example). Note that this weight-based total daily dose calculation and allocation is a starting point only and should be subsequently adjusted according to individualized insulin needs. The following provides an example total daily insulin dose calculation in a person recently diagnosed with T1D:

**Example 1:** RJ is a 60-kg woman recently diagnosed with T1D. It is decided that a total daily dose of 0.5 unit/kg/day is an appropriate starting point.

- **Total Daily Dose** = 60 kg × 0.5 unit/kg/day = *30 units/day*
- **Basal Dose** = 30 units/2 = *15 units of basal insulin daily*
- **Prandial Insulin** = Remaining 15 units/3 meals = *5 units of prandial insulin per meal*

Of note, there is no one gold standard method for initiating insulin in people with T1D. Although the previous example provides a starting point for insulin initiation, the weight-based dose calculation is an estimation of insulin needs only. For example, in people with T1D who are still in the honeymoon phase, lower weight-based doses of insulin may initially be needed until all endogenous insulin production has ceased. The basal and prandial insulin doses will inevitably require adjustment to meet individualized glycemic goals. Blood glucose monitoring data and CGM are important tools to evaluate an insulin regimen and inform insulin titration decisions. Ideally, people with T1D will learn to count carbohydrates and adjust insulin doses based on carbohydrate intake and also will utilize insulin correction doses to correct for residual hyperglycemia before meals and at bedtime. In the short term, however, fixed-dose prandial insulin can be used effectively until the patient is able to correctly count carbohydrates and adjust insulin doses based on meal content. Fixed dosing may also be a safer strategy in patients with limited self-care capabilities, such as those unable to reliably count carbohydrates. The following section provides specific information on establishing an insulin-to-carbohydrate (I:C) ratio.

## Insulin-to-Carbohydrate (I:C) Ratios

Ideally, prandial (mealtime) insulin doses are calculated in people with T1D to cover the amount of carbohydrate to be consumed. A typical ballpark I:C ratio in someone with T1D is 1:10 (1 unit of prandial insulin to cover 10 g of carbohydrate) or 1:15. These are estimates, however, and each person's needs vary. For people taking RAAs to cover meals, the "500 Rule" provides a reasonable initial estimate for determining a person's I:C ratio. To use the 500 Rule, the current total daily dose of insulin is simply divided into 500 to determine an estimated I:C ratio.

**Example 2:** SR, a man with T1D, is currently taking 30 units of U-100 insulin glargine once daily and a total of 20 units of insulin aspart divided among breakfast, lunch, and dinner. His total daily insulin dose is 50 units. SR would like to begin adjusting his mealtime insulin doses using an I:C ratio.

- **The 500 Rule:** 500/total daily insulin dose = 500/50 = 10
- **Interpretation:** 1 unit of insulin aspart will cover ~10 g of carbohydrate consumed with meals.
- **Application:** SR is planning to consume 40 g of carbohydrate at lunch. Using his estimated I:C ratio, he will inject 4 units of insulin aspart before the meal. SR was advised to check his blood glucose before the meal and 2 h after the meal to assess and reevaluate the appropriateness of his I:C ratio estimate.

## Correction Doses

Correction doses are important when blood glucose levels are unexpectedly elevated. A correction factor is ultimately used to correct for a blood glucose reading in the hyperglycemic range before meals or at bedtime, as examples. The "1800 Rule" is another simple calculation that can be used in people using RAAs at meals. The calculation estimates how far 1 unit of rapid-acting insulin will drop a person's blood glucose. To use the 1800 Rule, the number 1,800 is divided by the total daily dose of insulin to determine the individual's correction factor. The following example shows how to use the 1800 Rule to estimate a correction factor:

**Example 3:** MJ is currently taking 30 units of U-100 insulin glargine once daily and an average total of 30 units of insulin aspart divided among breakfast, lunch, and dinner after recently implementing an I:C ratio of 1:10. His total daily insulin dose is ~60 units. MJ would now like to determine his correction factor to better control his blood glucose throughout the day.

- **The 1800 Rule:** 1,800/total daily insulin dose = 1,800/60 = 30
- **Interpretation:** 1 unit of insulin aspart will drop MJ's blood glucose by an estimated 30 mg/dL.
- **Application:** MJ is about to consume 40 g of carbohydrate at lunch. His premeal blood glucose reading is 160 mg/dL (his goal premeal blood glucose is 100 mg/dL). Using his I:C ratio, he will administer 4 units to cover carbohydrates, and using his correction factor, he will administer an additional 2 units of insulin to account for the 60 mg/dL he is above his target premeal blood glucose. In total, MJ will administer 6 units of insulin aspart before lunch.

## *Ongoing Insulin Adjustment in T1D*

Although a variety of tools and estimates can be used to initiate and titrate insulin in people with T1D, the job of optimizing insulin therapy is an ongoing and iterative process. Insulin needs can and will change based on numerous factors. Illness, stress, diet, physical activity, and even the changing of the seasons can have drastic effects on glycemic control and insulin needs. Using information obtained from blood glucose monitoring and CGM can be extremely valuable in pinpointing glycemic trends and making adjustments to diet, physical activity, or insulin doses to improve glucose control. People with T1D should be encouraged and empowered to take an active role in identifying trends and factors that affect their blood glucose to improve their glucose control and quality of life. For additional information and recommendations related to the overall management of people with T1D, please refer to the Association's Position Statement *Type 1 Diabetes Through the Life Span*.

## Type 2 Diabetes

The approach to insulin use in people with T2D is quite different from the approach taken in people with T1D. Although people with T1D initiate an intensive insulin regimen shortly after diagnosis, people with T2D can often be managed with noninsulin therapies for years before the addition of insulin is required to meet individualized glycemic goals. That said, many people with T2D can benefit from early basal insulin initiation, depending on individualized needs and preferences. Once people with T2D reach the point at which they are not achieving individualized glycemic goals despite the use of multiple noninsulin therapies, they may need to progress to use of injectable therapies. **Figure 10** provides recommendations from the 2018 American Diabetes Association/European Association for the Study of Diabetes (EASD) consensus report on the management of hyperglycemia in T2D regarding treatment intensification to injectable therapies. As highlighted in **Figure 10**, for people with T2D who have an elevated A1C despite dual or triple therapy, it is recommended that a GLP-1 receptor agonist be considered as the first injectable agent in most patients. Insulin is recommended as the first injectable in those with a very high A1C (>11%), those with symptoms or evidence of catabolism (e.g., weight loss, polyuria, polydipsia), or if a diagnosis of T1D is a possibility. The figure provides some guidance on the initiation and titration of basal insulin, inclusive of a recommended starting dose (10 units/day or 0.1–0.2 units/kg/day) and guidance on titration of the basal insulin to achieve an individualized fasting glucose target. If goal A1C is not met following basal insulin optimization and achievement of the target fasting glucose level, the addition of prandial insulin is recommended. Prandial insulin is recommended to be started at 4 units/day or 10% of the basal dose typically initiated once daily with the largest meal (or meal with the largest postprandial glucose excursion). The dose can be uptitrated by 1–2 units or 10–15% twice weekly, with dose reductions of 10–20% recommended in the presence of hypoglycemia. Depending on response, additional injections of prandial insulin can be added until individualized glycemic goals are achieved. Although **Figure 10** provides a framework for insulin initiation and titration in people with T2D, individual patient needs will differ, and strategies should be individualized to meet glycemic goals and minimize hypoglycemia. The 2018 American Diabetes Association/EASD consensus report provides additional guidance on managing concomitant oral glucose-lowering medications once injectable therapies are initiated (**Figure 11**).

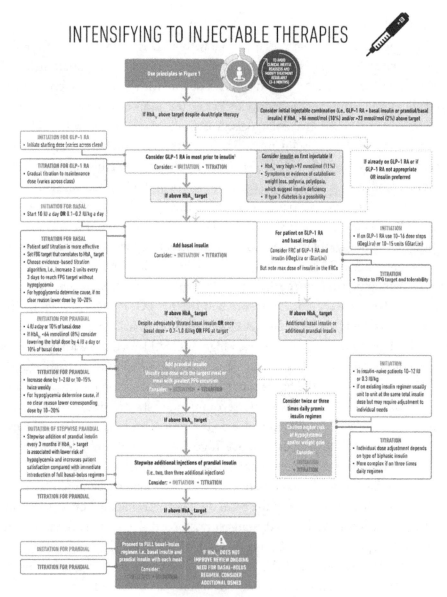

**Figure 10**—Combination injectable therapy for people with type 2 diabetes.

## CONSIDERING ORAL THERAPY IN COMBINATION WITH INJECTABLE THERAPIES

### METFORMIN

Continue treatment with metformin

### SGLT2i

If on SGLT2i, continue treatment
Consider adding SGLT2i if
- Established CVD
- If $HbA_{1c}$ above target or as weight reduction aid

### TZD[1]

Stop TZD when commencing insulin OR reduce dose

Beware
- DKA (euglycemic)
- Instruct on sick-day rules
- Do not down-titrate insulin over-aggressively

### SULFONYLUREA

If on SU, stop or reduce dose by 50% when basal insulin initiated

### DPP-4i

Stop DPP-4i if GLP-1 RA initiated

Consider stopping SU if prandial insulin initiated or on a premix regimen

1. Contraindicated in some countries, consider lower dose. This combination has a high risk of fluid retention and weight gain

**Figure 11**—Considering oral therapy in combination with injectable therapies.

# Sample Insulin Regimens

People with T1D will generally be on a regimen consisting of MDIs or use of an insulin pump, but insulin regimens can vary dramatically in people with T2D. The following discussion reviews select insulin regimens and their respective advantages and disadvantages.

## Two Injections per Day

*Regimen:* Mixed or premixed insulin: NPH plus a short- or rapid-acting insulin (**Figure 12** and **Figure 13**).

*Theory:* Postprandial glucose levels for the morning and evening meals are covered by short- or rapid-acting insulin; lunch and overnight glucose levels are covered by NPH.

*Advantage:* Provides some basal and mealtime coverage with only two injections per day.

*Disadvantages:* 1) NPH given at the evening meal peaks during the night and often does not last overnight until breakfast, leading to potential nocturnal hypoglycemia or high pre-breakfast glucose levels. 2) There is a lack of flexibility in dealing with midday glucose levels because the NPH dose and resultant action time are set at breakfast based on expectations of food and activity for the day. It would be unlikely that a patient with T1D could achieve adequate glucose control with this regimen.

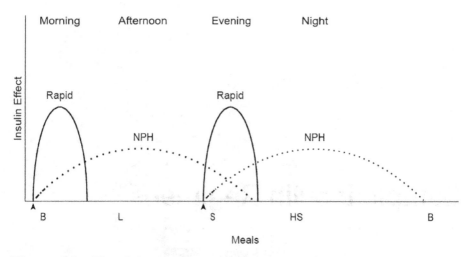

**Figure 12**—Two injections per day.

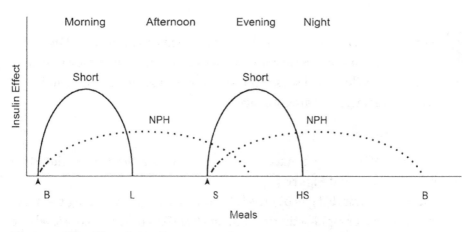

**Figure 13**—Two injections per day.

## Three Injections per Day

*Regimen:* Three injections per day using NPH and an RAA or short-acting insulin before breakfast, rapid-acting or short-acting insulin at the evening meal, and NPH at bedtime (**Figure 14** and **Figure 15**).

*Theory:* Same advantages as discussed for two injections per day, except that administering NPH at bedtime rather than at the evening meal may better control glucose levels overnight.

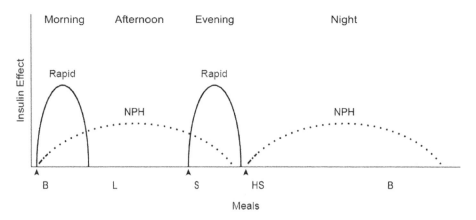

**Figure 14**—Three injections per day.

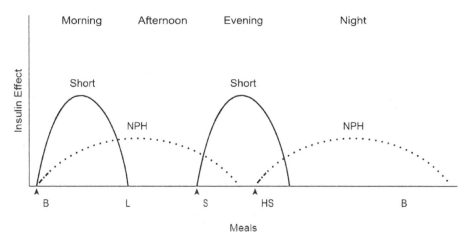

**Figure 15**—Three injections per day.

*Advantage:* Better overnight glucose control compared with a twice-daily premixed regimen.

*Disadvantage:* There is a lack of flexibility in dealing with midday glucose levels after lunch. Again, it would be unlikely that a patient with T1D could achieve adequate glucose control with this regimen.

## Four Injections per Day, Regimen 1

*Regimen:* Four injections per day using rapid-acting insulin analog plus twice-daily NPH or a long-acting insulin analog (**Figure 16** and **Figure 17**).

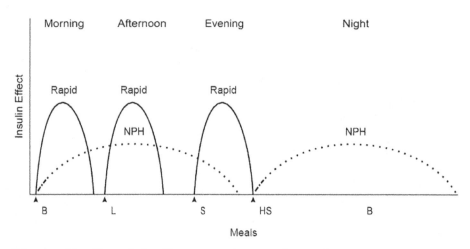

**Figure 16**—Four injections per day, regimen 1.

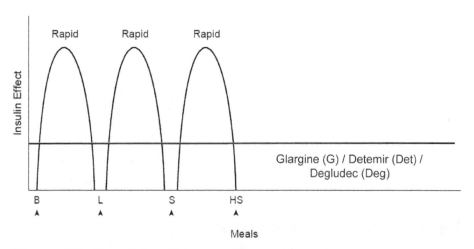

**Figure 17**—Four injections per day, regimen 1.

*Theory:* Two doses of NPH or one or two doses of long-acting insulin provide basal coverage during the day and overnight. Rapid-acting insulin covers postprandial glucose with each meal.

*Advantages:* Allows meal-to-meal adjustments of insulin dose based on preprandial glucose levels, carbohydrate intake, and activity and permits greater freedom of timing for meals.

*Disadvantages for NPH-containing regimen: 1)* NPH given in the evening peaks during the night and often does not last overnight until breakfast, leading to potential nocturnal hypoglycemia or high pre-breakfast glucose levels. 2) Initial injection at breakfast requires mixing the NPH and rapid insulins.

## Four Injections per Day, Regimen 2

*Regimen:* Four injections per day using short-acting insulin and twice-daily NPH or a long-acting insulin analog (**Figure 18** and **Figure 19**).

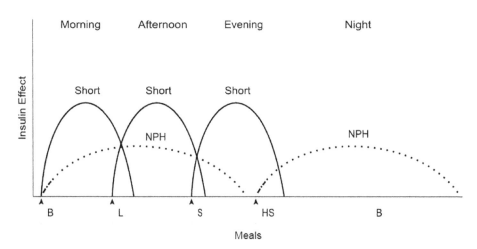

**Figure 18**—Four injections per day, regimen 2.

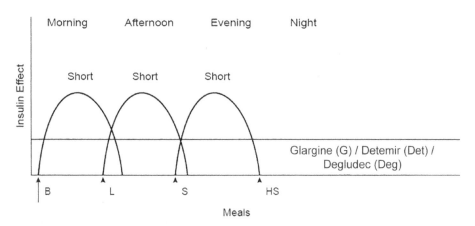

**Figure 19**—Four injections per day, regimen 2.

*Theory:* Short-acting insulin provides daytime and meal glucose control, and one dose of long-acting insulin analog or twice-daily NPH provides basal coverage during the day and overnight.

*Advantage:* Allows meal-to-meal adjustments of insulin based on preprandial glucose levels, carbohydrate intake, and activity.

*Disadvantage:* The long duration of regular insulin may lead to delayed (especially nocturnal) hypoglycemia.

# Troubleshooting Barriers to Insulin Use and Key Adverse Events

Although intensive (basal/bolus) insulin therapy is unmatched in terms of glucose-lowering potential, its use comes with risks of hypoglycemia, weight gain, and injection site reactions. Initiation of insulin therapy inherently comes with a requirement of more intensive medical oversight and training related to proper insulin use and administration. These considerations can lead to hesitance to initiate insulin on the part of both people with diabetes and healthcare providers alike.

## Barriers to Insulin Use in Type 2 Diabetes

Many people with T2D would achieve better glucose control with insulin, but the patient or the provider may resist beginning injections despite rising glycemic levels for fear of complicating the therapy or concerns regarding hypoglycemia. Education is the key to increasing provider knowledge and comfort with using insulin. Providers who are comfortable with insulin therapy are more apt to gain patient acceptance when insulin therapy is indicated. Patient education and positive support are key components to effective and safe use of insulin.

Suggestions to increase knowledge and acceptance of insulin therapy for patients with T2D include the following:

- Provide education and ensure understanding that the disease course includes progressive β-cell failure and that insulin therapy is generally an expected treatment of the condition, not a sign of failure on the part of the patient.
- Avoid using the prospect of insulin therapy as a threat to increase adherence to lifestyle change or other therapies.
- Reinforce the short-term benefits of improved glycemia, including decreased nocturia and improved energy levels.
- Reinforce or reintroduce information about the importance of controlling glucose levels that preserve the health and overall well-being and prevent long-term complications of kidneys, eyes, and the cardiovascular and nervous systems.
- Suggest that the patient try a bedtime injection routine of insulin glargine, detemir, degludec, or NPH for 1–2 months, and then plan to discuss whether the patient feels better and has more energy.
- Point out that newer needles make insulin therapy essentially painless and much more convenient than before, and offer alternatives to syringes, such as insulin pens.
- Provide or refer the patient for diabetes self-management education on handling and filling syringes, making injections as comfortable as possible, and for ongoing self-management support.

## Hypoglycemia

Hypoglycemia is the most common and serious adverse event associated with insulin use. Hypoglycemia is defined generally as a blood glucose value ≤70 mg/dL, with lower blood glucose levels associated with worsening hypoglycemic symptoms. Hypoglycemia is much more common with the use of prandial insulin products. Careful and methodic titration of basal insulin products can minimize hypoglycemia risk, although overbasalization can contribute to hypoglycemic events. If overbasalization is suspected, blood glucose testing overnight may be warranted to determine whether the basal insulin is precipitously dropping the blood glucose overnight. Because people with T1D are managed with intensive insulin regimens, they are generally at greater risk for hypoglycemia. That said, some people with T2D also receive intensive insulin therapy and should be considered high risk for hypoglycemic events, particularly when insulin is used in combination with sulfonylureas or other insulin secretagogue medications. Use of insulin in combination with insulin sensitizers (such as thiazolidinediones) may also increase risk.

All people who use insulin should be counseled regarding the signs, symptoms, and proper treatment of hypoglycemia. Although not exhaustive, **Table 6** provides a list of potential hypoglycemic symptoms. Mild hypoglycemia can be treated by following the "rule of 15": treat with 15 g carbohydrate, wait 15 min, and then check the blood glucose level. If after 15 min the blood glucose remains <70 mg/dL, another 15 g of carbohydrate should be consumed. Once the blood glucose is normalized, a snack or meal including complex carbohydrates and protein should be consumed to prevent a secondary hypoglycemic episode. When a severe hypoglycemic event occurs and glucose cannot be delivered orally, SC or IM glucagon use is indicated. The Association's *Standards of Medical Care in Diabetes* recommend that glucagon be prescribed to individuals at significant risk of severe hypoglycemia, which would include people who use prandial insulin products.

### Table 6—Symptoms of Hypoglycemia

- Shakiness
- Nervousness or anxiety
- Sweating, chills, or clamminess
- Irritability or impatience
- Confusion, including delirium
- Rapid or fast heartbeat
- Lightheadedness or dizziness
- Hunger and nausea
- Sleepiness
- Blurred or impaired vision
- Tingling or numbness in the lips or tongue
- Headaches
- Weakness or fatigue
- Anger, stubbornness, or sadness
- Lack of coordination
- Nightmares
- Seizures
- Unconsciousness

## Hypoglycemia Unawareness

Some patients lose their ability to recognize normal warning symptoms of hypoglycemia, or the symptoms are blunted or absent. These patients are at high risk to experience severe hypoglycemia. Hypoglycemia unawareness develops more commonly in patients with T1D who have frequent hypoglycemic episodes and have had diabetes for many years. Preventing hypoglycemia can reverse hypoglycemia unawareness. The Association states that patients with hypoglycemia unawareness who experience one or more severe hypoglycemic events may benefit from at least short-term relaxation of glycemic targets so that their awareness and counter-regulation can be improved. Hypoglycemia awareness training also can improve patient recognition of early manifestations of hypoglycemia and prevent episodes of severe hypoglycemia. Patients with hypoglycemia unawareness are particularly suitable candidates for use of CGM to detect and prevent hypoglycemic events. Patients should additionally receive education about prevention and safety, including more frequent SMBG, particularly before driving or other potentially dangerous activities. Patients should receive a prescription for glucagon, with appropriate counseling and education on use provided to the patient and their family members or caregivers.

## Weight Gain

Weight gain is associated with insulin use and is observed as improvements in glycemic control are achieved. As glycemic control improves, glucose is utilized by the tissues instead of being lost in the urine, thus resulting in weight gain. Although weight gain is initially viewed as desirable in people with T1D because of the weight loss experienced secondary to glucosuria and catabolism that is frequently present at the time of diagnosis, intensive insulin therapy can result in undesirable weight gain over time. Indeed, some patients with T1D may even underdose insulin to avoid weight gain. For those with T2D, who often struggle with overweight and obesity, insulin therapy can further contribute to weight gain. Use of prandial insulin in people with T2D generally contributes to more weight gain than the use of basal insulin products alone. Both hypoglycemia treatment and possibly increased caloric intake in defense against hypoglycemia can result in weight gain. People starting insulin therapy should be informed of the potential for weight gain and be encouraged to implement healthy lifestyle measures to minimize insulin-induced weight gain. In people with T2D, adjunctive antihyperglycemic agents, such as GLP-1 receptor agonists, SGLT2 inhibitors, and pramlintide, can be used for their insulin-sparing and weight-mitigating effects. Medications approved by the FDA for weight loss can also be considered.

## Adjustments for Physical Activity

When initiating an exercise routine, it can be useful to encourage people with diabetes to exercise at the same time every day, for the same duration, and at the same intensity, to facilitate consistent therapy adjustments that will reduce the risk of severe hypoglycemia, particularly for patients with T1D. In addition, SMBG before and after exercise will help identify necessary changes in food or insulin intake and educate the patient about his or her individual glycemic response to particular physical activities. Once patients understand how to adjust their insulin and food intake in relation to exercise, they will be better able to anticipate the adjustments needed for varying types and times of physical activity.

The following guidelines apply primarily to patients with T1D; however, if a person with T2D experiences exercise-induced hypoglycemia, these same guidelines can be helpful:

- When the patient plans to exercise after a meal, begin by cutting the meal-related rapid- or short-acting insulin dose. If the patient is unfamiliar with the glycemic effect of a given activity and the activity is more strenuous, reduce the dose by half. Use SMBG results to determine whether the lowered dose resulted in hyperglycemia, glucose within the target range (80–130 mg/dL), or hypoglycemia. If needed, adjust up or down by 3% of total daily insulin requirements to prepare for a similar bout of exercise (i.e., similar in timing, duration, intensity).
- When the patient plans to exercise before eating, he or she may need to eat supplementary carbohydrates. This is a simpler option than reducing the prandial insulin dose before a meal.

# Patient Education and Resources

Perhaps the most important aspect of diabetes care is the patient–healthcare provider relationship. One essential element of this partnership is patient education. Encourage your patients to learn all they can about how to successfully self-manage their diabetes, including appropriate insulin dose adjustments in response to SMBG results.

Stress to your patients that testing, recordkeeping, healthy eating, and engaging in physical activity are for their benefit. Healthy living with diabetes is largely driven by a patient's efforts at diabetes self-management.

A wide variety of patient education materials are available from the American Diabetes Association. Your patients can reach the American Diabetes Association Call Center at 1-800-DIABETES and visit the American Diabetes Association website at www.diabetes.org.

The American Diabetes Association has a wide variety of medical management publications for healthcare professionals, such as the following books:

- *American Diabetes Association Guide to Nutrition Therapy for Diabetes*, 3rd edition
- *American Diabetes Association/JDRF Type 1 Diabetes Sourcebook*
- *Approaches to Behavior*
- *Atypical Diabetes*

- *Clinical Care of the Diabetic Foot*, 3rd edition
- *Complementary and Alternative Medicine Supplement Use in People with Diabetes: A Clinician's Guide*
- *Complete Nurse's Guide to Diabetes*, 3rd edition
- *Diabetes Case Studies*
- *Diabetes Management in Long-Term Settings*
- *Diabetes Risks from Prescription and Nonprescription Drugs*
- *Diabetes Technology*
- *Exercise and Diabetes*
- *Guide to Medications for the Treatment of Diabetes Mellitus*
- *Hypoglycemia in Diabetes*, 3rd edition
- *Intensive Diabetes Management*, 6th edition
- *Managing Diabetes and Hyperglycemia in the Hospital Setting*
- *Medical Management of Pregnancy Complicated by Diabetes*, 6th edition
- *Medical Management of Type 1 Diabetes*, 7th edition
- *Medical Management of Type 2 Diabetes*, 7th edition
- *Meeting the American Diabetes Association Standards of Care*, 2nd edition
- *Psychosocial Care for People with Diabetes*
- *Putting Your Patients on the Pump*, 2nd edition
- *Teens with Diabetes: A Clinician's Guide*
- *Therapy for Diabetes Mellitus and Related Disorders*, 6th edition

For more information on these and other professional titles published by the American Diabetes Association:

- Visit the American Diabetes Association online bookstore at www.shopdiabetes.org
- Call 1-800-232-6733
- Visit any nationwide bookseller

## Appendix 1 — Typical Development and Diabetes Demands and Priorities Across Childhood

| Ages and Corresponding Developmental Level | Typical Developmental Tasks | T1D Management Priorities (and Person Responsible) | Family Considerations due to Presence of T1D |
|---|---|---|---|
| 0–2 years; infancy and start of toddlerhood | Attachment and development of trusting bond with caregivers<br><br>Physical development and reaching milestones of first words and walking | Reduction of wide fluctuations in glucose levels (caregiver)<br><br>Prevention of hypoglycemia (caregiver) | Vigilance in identifying child symptoms of hypo- and hyperglycemia<br><br>Coping with stress associated with management and additional responsibilities |
| 2–6 years; end of toddlerhood through early childhood | Often begin formal schooling — preschool to elementary school<br><br>Separating from caregivers for activities<br><br>Physical growth with interests in exploring new challenges and activities | Reduction of wide fluctuations in glucose levels (caregiver, school personnel)<br><br>Prevention of hypoglycemia (caregivers, school personnel)<br><br>Trusting others to help with diabetes management (child) | Continued vigilance in identifying child symptoms<br><br>Communicating and planning for monitoring when not with child; coping with stress<br><br>Close monitoring of food intake and adjustments for variable appetites |
| 7–11 years; late childhood | Developing skills in physical, social, and academic areas<br><br>Gaining more autonomy from primary caregivers, yet still very reliant on caregiver supervision and planning<br><br>Often engaging in team activities that promote sharing and understanding views of others | Sharing in the identification of symptoms of hypo- and hyperglycemia (child and caregiver)<br><br>Treating hypoglycemia and carrying supplies (child with planning/supervision from adults)<br><br>Developing sense of problem solving and flexibility with regimen if plans or activities change (child with guidance/modeling from caregiver) | Teaching child symptoms of hyperglycemia and hypoglycemia<br><br>Teaching basics of diabetes management and treatment<br><br>Praising conduct of management tasks |

*(Continued)*

## Appendix 1 –(Continued)

| Ages and Corresponding Developmental Level | Typical Developmental Tasks | T1D Management Priorities (and Person Responsible) | Family Considerations due to Presence of T1D |
|---|---|---|---|
| | | | Modeling problem solving when new diabetes problems arise |
| | | | Helping teach child to disclose to others about diabetes |
| | | | Coping with stress and new challenges of complex schedules and eating patterns |
| 12–15 years; early adolescence | Managing changes with body | More decision making about diabetes management and regimen changes (teen) | Coping with common increase in conflict about diabetes management |
| | Attempts at "fitting in" with peer groups; peers becoming larger influence on behavior | Expectation to monitor and be vigilant about glucose excursions when away from primary caregivers (teen) | Developing new forms of monitoring and communicating about diabetes |
| | Developing stronger sense of self and identity | Disclose to others about diabetes for safety (teen) | Supervising enough but attempting to support growing autonomy in teen |
| | Desiring less guidance and supervision from caregivers, yet still needing it | | |
| 16–19 years; late adolescence | Expansion of networks and activities | Increasing autonomy for many management tasks (teen) | Balancing need for supervision and guidance with less face-to-face time with teen and more teen autonomy |
| | Increased thinking and worries about what is next | Diminishing seeking of guidance and supervision from caregivers (teens) | Modeling positive decision making about diabetes and life choices |
| | Expectation to make decisions based on interests and opportunities | Discussions about transition to different diabetes care providers (teens, care team, and caregivers) | Creating scaffolding for transition with diabetes and next phase of life |

T1D, type 1 diabetes.

*Source:* Chiang JL, Maahs DM, Garvey KC, Hood KK, Laffel LM, Weinzimer SA, Wolfsdorf JI, Schatz D. Type 1 diabetes in children and adolescents: A position statement by the American Diabetes Association. *Diabetes Care* 2018; 41(9):2026–2044.

## Appendix 2—Sample Blood Glucose Log

| Date | Time | Breakfast | Medicine/Comment | Time | Lunch | Medicine/Comment | Time | Dinner | Medicine/Comment | Time | Snack/Other | Medicine/Comment |
|---|---|---|---|---|---|---|---|---|---|---|---|---|
| | | | | | | | | | | | | |
| | | | | | | | | | | | | |
| | | | | | | | | | | | | |
| | | | | | | | | | | | | |
| | | | | | | | | | | | | |
| | | | | | | | | | | | | |
| | | | | | | | | | | | | |

# Index

**Note:** Page numbers followed by an *f* refer to figures. Page numbers followed by a *t* refer to tables. Page numbers in **bold** indicate an in-depth discussion.

## A

A1C (hemoglobin $A_{1c}$), 2
    premixed insulin products, 15
    type 1 diabetes (T1D), 28, 29
    type 2 diabetes (T2D), 33, 34*f*, 35*f*
absorption, insulin, 23–24
adipose, 1, 23
Admelog, 10
Afrezza (inhalable human insulin powder), 8*t*, 10–11, 10*f*, 18*t*
albumin, 12
amino acid sequence, 4
aspart, 7, 8*t*, 10, 15, 16*t*, 18, 21

## B

Basaglar, 12
basal insulin, 3
   hypoglycemia, 44
   type 1 diabetes (T1D), 30
   type 2 diabetes (T2D), 33, 34*f*
   weight gain, 46

## C

carbohydrates
   hypoglycemia, 45
   insulin-to-carbohydrate ratio (I:C), 31
   metabolism, 3
   physical activity, 47
   rapid-acting analogs (RAAs), 28
   type 1 diabetes (T1D), 21, 30
β-cells
   type 1 diabetes (T1D), 27
   type 2 diabetes (T2D), 3–4, 44
chronic obstructive pulmonary disease, 11
continuous glucose monitor (CGM)
   CSII, 20
   hypoglycemia, 46
   type 1 diabetes (T1D), 30, 32
continuous subcutaneous insulin infusion (CSII, insulin pump),
  **20–22,** 21*f,* 22*f,* 28, 29, 37
correction doses, type 1 diabetes (T1D), 31–32
cortisol, 4*f*

## D

dawn phenomenon, 4*f*
degludec (U-100,U-200), 8–10, 8*t,* **13–14,** 15, 16*t,* 18, 20, 44

detemir, **12–13,** 18, 44
Diabetes Control and Complications Trial (DCCT), 28
DPP-4i, 35*f*

## E

education, **49–50,** 51*t*–53*t*
1800 Rule, 31–32
euglycemia, 3
European Association for the Study of Diabetes (EASD), 33

## F

fasting plasma glucose (FPG), 27, 34*f*
Fiasp (faster acting insulin aspart product), 8*t*, 10, 18
500 Rule, 31
Food and Drug Administration (FDA), 8–10
four injections per day, **39–42,** 40*f,* 41*f*

## G

glargine (U-100), 8*t*, 9*f,* **12,** 18, 31, 32
glargine (U-300), 9*f,* **13,** 18, 20
glucagon, 45
glucagon-like peptide 1 receptor agonists (GLP-1 receptor agonists), 15
    type 2 diabetes (T2D), 33, 34*f,* 35*f*
    weight gain, 47
glulisine, 7, 8*t,* 9, 18, 21
growth hormone, 4*f*

## H

Humalog, 10
hyperglycemia, 3
    physical activity, 47
    type 1 diabetes (T1D), 30

hypoglycemia, 1
   four injections per day, 42
   insulin degludec, 14
   insulin glargine (U-300), 13
   intramuscular administration (IM), 22
   neutral protamine Hagedorn (NPH), 11
   physical activity, 47
   symptoms, 45*t*
   three injections per day, 41
   type 1 diabetes (T1D), 29, **44–45**
   type 2 diabetes (T2D), 33, 34*f,* 45
   U-100, 12
   unawareness, **46**
   weight gain, **46**

# I

injection therapies, **22–23,** 23*f*
   four injections per day, **39–42,** 40*f,* 41*f*
   three injections per day, **38–39,** 39*f*
   two injections per day, **37,** 38*f*
   type 2 diabetes (T2D), 33, 34*f,* 35*f*
insulin, 4, 5*f*
   absorption, **23–24**
   administration and use, **17–25,** 18*t*
   available products, **7–15,** 16*t,* 18*t*
   basic pharmacology, **3–5**
   correction doses, 31–32
   delivery methods, 17–22, 19*f,* 21*f,* 22*f*
   education, **49–50,** 51*t*–53*t*
   injection therapies, 22–23, 23*f*
      four injections per day, **39–42,** 40*f,* 41*f*
      three injections per day, **38–39,** 39*f*
      two injections per day, **37,** 38*f*

recommended use, **27–32**
storage of, 18*t*, **25**
weight gain, 46–47
insulin aspart, 7, 8*t*, 10, 15, 16*t*, 18, 21
insulin degludec (U-100, U-200), 8–10, 8*t*, **13–14,** 15, 16*t*, 18, 20, 44
insulin detemir, **12–13,** 18, 44
insulin glargine (U-100), 8*t*, 9*f*, **12,** 18, 31, 32
insulin glargine (U-300), 9*f*, **13,** 18, 20
insulin glulisine, 7, 8*t*, 18, 21
insulin lispro, 7, 8, 8*t*, 15, 16*t*, 18, 21
insulin pump (continuous subcutaneous insulin infusion), 20–22, 21*f*, 22*f*, 28, 29, 37
insulin sensitizers, 45
insulin-to-carbohydrate ratio (I:C), **31**
intermediate-acting insulin, 8*t*, **11–12**
intramuscular administration (IM), 22–23
islets of Langerhans, 3
isophane, 8*t*, 11–12

## L

Lantus, 12
lipids, 3
lipoatrophy, 23
lipohypertrophy, 23–24
lispro, 7, 8, 8*t*, 15, 16*t*, 18, 21
long-acting insulin, **12–15,** 25, 28
lysine, 14

## M

metformin, 35*f*
multiple daily injections (MDIs), 28, 37

## N

neutral protamine Hagedorn (NPH), 8*t*, **11–12**
    four injections per day, 39–42, 40*f*
    storage, 25
    three injections per day, 38–39, 39*f*
    two injections per day, 37, 38*f*
    type 2 diabetes (T2D), 44
niacinamide, 10
NovoLog, 10

## O

obesity, 23
overdose, 14

## P

pens, 18*t*, 19*f*, **20**, 25, 44
phenol, 14
physical activity, **47**
polydipsia, 33, 34*f*
polyuria, 33, 34*f*
pramlintide, 47
prandial insulin
    hypoglycemia, 44
    physical activity, 47
    type 1 diabetes (T1D), 30
    type 2 diabetes (T2D), 33, 34*f*
premixed insulin products, **15**, 16*t*
protamine, 11
protein, 3

## R

rapid-acting analogs (RAAs), **7–11**, 8*t*, 9*f*
    CSII, 21

four injections per day, 39–41, 40f
premixed insulin products, 15, 16t
storage, 25
three injections per day, 38–39
two injections per day, 37, 38f
type 1 diabetes (T1D), 28, 31
recombinant DNA, 4
regular human insulin (RHI), 8, 8t, 11, 18
ReliOn, 11, 12
RHI (regular human insulin), 8, 8t, 11, 18

# S

self-monitoring of blood glucose (SMBG), 2
   education, 49
   hypoglycemia, 46
   physical activity, 47
SGLT2i, 35f, 47
short-acting insulin, 8t, **11**
   four injections per day, 41–42, 41f
   storage, 25
   three injections per day, 38–39
   two injections per day, 37, 38f
subcutaneous administration (SC)
   CSII, 20
   Fiasp, 10
   insulin absorption, 23–24
   insulin degludec (U-100), 14
   insulin degludec (U-200), 14
   insulin glargine (U-100), 31
   insulin lispro, 8
   RHI, 11
sulfonylurea (SU), 35f, 45
syringes, 19f, **20**
   type 2 diabetes (T2D), 44

# T

thiazolidinediones, 45
three injections per day, **38–39**, 39f
threonine, 12
two injections per day, **37**, 38f
type 1 diabetes (T1D), 1, 2
- CSII, 20–21
- 1800 Rule, 31–32
- Fiasp, 10
- glucose, 3
- glycemic goals, **28–29**, 29t
- hypoglycemia, 44–45
    - unawareness, 46
- inhalable human insulin powder, 10
- insulin
    - absorption, 24
    - correction doses, **31–32**
    - initiation, **30–31**
    - ongoing adjustment, 32
    - recommended use, **27–32**
- physical activity, 47
- weight gain, 46–47

type 2 diabetes (T2D), 1, 2
- β-cells, 3–4
- Fiasp, 10
- hypoglycemia, 45
- inhalable human insulin powder, 10
- injection therapies, 33, 34f, 35f
    - three injections per day, 38–39, 39f
- insulin
    - absorption, 24
    - barriers, **43–44**
    - recommended use, **33**, 34f, 35f

physical activity, 47
regular insulin (U-500), 15
weight gain, 46–47
TZD, 35*f*

## U

U-500 (regular insulin), 7, 8*t*, **14–15**, 18

## V

V-Go patch pump, 20
vials, **20**, 25

## W

weight gain
   insulin, **46–47**
   premixed insulin products, 15
   type 1 diabetes (T1D), 1, 46–47
   type 2 diabetes (T2D), 46–47
weight loss, type 2 diabetes (T2D), 33, 34*f*